Best of Therapie

Mit „Best of Therapie" zeichnet Springer die besten Masterarbeiten aus den Bereichen Ergotherapie, Logopädie und Physiotherapie aus. Inhalte aus den etablierten Bereichen der Therapiewissenschaft, Pädagogik, des Gesundheitsmanagements und der Grundlagenforschung finden hier eine geeignete Plattform. Die mit Bestnote ausgezeichneten Arbeiten wurden durch Gutachter empfohlen und behandeln aktuelle Themen rund um die Therapiewissenschaften im Gesundheitswesen.
Die Reihe wendet sich an Praktiker und Wissenschaftler gleichermaßen und soll insbesondere auch Nachwuchswissenschaftlern Orientierung geben.

Weitere Bände in der Reihe http://www.springer.com/series/15357

Sarah Klamroth

Perturbation Treadmill Training in Parkinson's Disease

A Novel Approach for Neurological Rehabilitation

With a preface by Prof. Dr. Klaus Pfeifer and Dr. Simon Steib

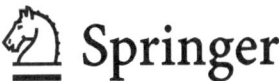 Springer

Sarah Klamroth
Erlangen, Germany

Best of Therapie
ISBN 978-3-658-20542-3   ISBN 978-3-658-20543-0   (eBook)
https://doi.org/10.1007/978-3-658-20543-0

Library of Congress Control Number: 2017963265

Printed on acid-free paper

This Springer imprint is published by Springer Nature
The registered company is Springer Fachmedien Wiesbaden GmbH
The registered company address is: Abraham-Lincoln-Str. 46, 65189 Wiesbaden, Germany

Preface

The master thesis by Sarah Klamroth titled *Acute effects of a novel treadmill device on gait and postural control in persons with Parkinson's disease* addresses a highly relevant issue in the field of neurological rehabilitation with a specific focus on the sensorimotor control system. The thesis was part of a larger interdisciplinary research project (EFI – Emerging Fields Initiative of the Friedrich-Alexander-University Erlangen-Nürnberg), which investigated a novel type of treadmill training that applies additional perturbations to the walking surface. Within this research cooperation, Ms. Klamroth conducted a separate experimental study to analyze the short-term motor adaptations in gait and postural control in Parkinson patients after a single session of perturbation treadmill training. A secondary aim of the study was to identify predictors which might explain differences in motor adaptations across participants. This work provides a good theoretical background for the development of perturbation treadmill training, and investigates the short-term motor adaptations to this novel training device in patients with Parkinson's Disease. The thesis is written in article style for publication in an international peer-reviewed journal.

The high quality of this master thesis is seen especially in the study design, the complex data analysis and in the extensive interpretation of the results. The work also benefits from Sarah Klamroth's practical skills and theoretical background as a physical therapist. Her experience in treating Parkinson patients was not only beneficial for conducting the treadmill training, but is also reflected in the discussion section which addresses the relevance and transfer of her findings. Finally, the publication of this work in the high-ranking international journal *Gait & Posture* underpins the relevance of the addressed topic and the excellent quality of this master thesis.

Prof. Dr. Klaus Pfeifer and Dr. Simon Steib

Institute Profile

The Department of Sport Science and Sport (DSS) at the Friedrich-Alexander-University (FAU) Erlangen-Nürnberg is one of the leading institutions for sport science in Germany. In recent years it has established itself as an international scientific center for competence in *Health and Physical Activity*. The main focus of the DSS lies in human movement within sport as well as other fields, primarily from a sport science perspective but also including other related research areas. The main topic *Health and Physical Activity* is covered by the four divisions of the DSS: *Physical Activity and Public Health, Exercise and Health, Education in Sport,* and *Sport and Exercise Medicine*, which are all mutually connected. In order to facilitate activities incorporating research, teaching and University Sports, the DSS integrates the *University Sports* as a fifth division.

The Division of *Exercise and Health* (Chair: Prof. Dr. Klaus Pfeifer) investigates the health-related potential of physical activity and exercise. Here, possibilities for the enhancement of movement related health competence focus on the spectrum between physiological adaptations and individual health behavior. Therefore, questions related to baseline conditions and assessment methods as well as to the conceptualization, implementation and evaluation of respective interventions are addressed. In the context of interdisciplinary applied projects, there are several close cooperations with physicians, psychologists, teachers, physiotherapists, gerontologists and key stakeholders in the health sector. The field of Exercise and Health focuses primarily on three research topics: 1) Physical Activity Promotion and Health Research, 2) Exercise Therapy and Motor Control, 3) Digitized Exercise Therapy and Physical Activity Promotion. The master thesis by Sarah Klamroth investigated motor adaptations in people with Parkinson's Disease after a specific type of exercise therapy (treadmill training). This therefore belongs to the research topic of *Exercise Therapy and Motor Control* in the division of *Exercise and Health*.

The DSS pursues an integrative-cooperative research approach built on inter- and transdisciplinary knowledge transfer between the different fields of *Physical Activity and Health*. The main goal is to generate sport scientific knowledge that is practically useful, and to develop, implement and evaluate concepts in the field of Physical Activity and Health. In order to reach this goal, the four divisions within the DSS strongly collaborate with players in the health sector (e.g. rehabilitation clinics, health insurance companies, german pension insurance), in the education and research system (e.g. Department of Education and Cultural Affairs, cooperating universities), in the organized sport sector (e.g. DOSB – Deutscher Olympischer Sportbund), and with stakeholders in economy and industry (e.g. sporting goods manufacturers).

Students enrolled in one of the programs offered by the DSS also benefit from current research activities and findings. At the moment, the DSS offers the following programs: a Bachelor in Sport Science (extra-occupational); an international sport science Masters in Physical Activity and Health; a PhD program in Physical Activity and Health; and Physical Education Teaching Programs (for all kinds of german schools). All studies at the DSS aim for developing professional capabilities by enabling students to cope with complex situations in the professional fields related to sport, physical activity and health.

Prof. Dr. Klaus Pfeifer

Acknowledgements

I would like to thank all the people who contributed in some way to the work described in this master thesis.

At first, I like to express my gratitude to my supervisors Dr. Simon Steib und Prof. Dr. Klaus Pfeifer for her inspiring feedback and support through the process of researching and writing this thesis. I am very thankful that my supervisors made it possible that my master thesis could be part of a larger cooperative research project (EFI-Moves) of the Friedrich-Alexander-University Erlangen – Nürnberg.

Furthermore, I would like to acknowledge the research team of the EFI-Moves project for the great cooperation and support. My special thanks to Dr. Heiko Gassner, Dr. Jochen Klucken and Prof. Dr. Jürgen Winkler from the University Hospital Erlangen, and Prof. Dr. Björn Eskofier from the Pattern Recognition Lab of the Friedrich-Alexander-University Erlangen – Nürnberg.

Also, I like to thank the participants in my experimental study, who have willingly shared their precious time. This study would not have been possible without their participation.

Finally, I like to thank my family and my friends for their patience and for keeping me harmonious through the process of researching and writing this thesis.

Sarah Klamroth

Table of Contents

List of Figures and Tables

Abstract

Objective: Investigation of acute adaptations in gait and postural control in individuals with Parkinson's disease after a single session of perturbational treadmill training.

Design: Randomized controlled trial.

Setting. University laboratory for research and promotion of physical activity.

Subjects: People with Parkinson's disease (n=39) in stage 1 to 3 of the Hoehn and Yahr Scale.

Intervention: All participants received a single treadmill training session. The experimental group (n=19) walked with perturbations produced by small three-dimensional tilting movements of the belt which simulate an uneven surface. The control group (n=20) performed treadmill training without additional perturbations.

Main measures: Primary measures were self-selected comfortable overground walking speed (10-Meter-Walk-Test) and center of pressure sway velocity (vCOP) and –sway area (aCOP). Secondary measures were spatiotemporal gait parameters during treadmill walking.

Results: The experimental group significantly improved in overground walking speed after intervention, compared to the control group (p = .014; ES = +0.41). By contrast, postural control measures did not differ significantly between groups after intervention. While treadmill walking, only the experimental group significantly reduced measures of gait variability. Walking without handrail support during perturbations predicted significant improvements in step time symmetry (p = .029; ES = -0.36) and variability of cadence (p = .002; ES = -0.52). More disabled patients significantly improved in overground walking speed (p = .016; ES = +0.40) and stance phase symmetry (p = .011; ES = -0.42) if they trained with perturbations.

Conclusions: One session of perturbational treadmill training led to beneficial acute adaptations in gait performance but not in postural control.

1 Introduction

Parkinson's disease (PD) is a progressive neurological disorder with a growing worldwide prevalence[1] and associated rising health costs in the future[2]. The disease is characterized mainly by four cardinal motor symptoms: resting tremor, bradykinesia, rigidity and postural instability.[3] These symptoms often cause gait disturbances, such as reduced gait speed and shortened step length, leading to disability and reduced quality of life.[4,5]

Within the past years treadmill training has become an important therapeutic tool in neurologic rehabilitation.[6–12] People with PD significantly improved their gait speed, step length and walking distance after regular treadmill training.[13] A few trials also investigated the acute adaptations in this population after a single treadmill session and showed improvements in gait speed, stride length and double stance phase.[14–16]

While previous studies on treadmill training mainly varied walking speed[15,17] and body-weight support[14,18,19], recent trials focused on explorative designs where participants are perturbed during treadmill walking. Such interventions included bilateral separated treadmill walking[20,21] which manipulates participants' gait symmetry, perturbation of synchronized movements by applying specific forces to the lower limbs[22,23], visual-induced perturbations by manipulating the virtual environment[24,25], and treadmill training which provokes slips or trips of participants by sudden medio-lateral[26–28] or anterior-posterior[29–39] movements of the belt. Although these types of perturbations were very heterogeneous, all of them represented an additional postural challenge during treadmill walking.

Especially in PD, combining treadmill walking with balance training may enhance the beneficial effects of conventional treadmill training[13], since studies have suggested that highly challenging balance exercises can counteract postural instability in PD[40]. Thus a novel treadmill device (Zebris medical GmbH, H/P cosmos GmbH) was developed, with the purpose of applying additional perturbations during walking. To challenge participants' postural control, pneumatic actuators below the treadmill constantly induce small three-dimensional tilting movements. The primary purpose of this study was to examine acute adaptations in gait and postural control in individuals with PD after a single training session on the novel treadmill device. A secondary aim was to identify specific predictors which might explain differences in adaptations across participants.

2 Methods

2.1 Design and Participants

From June 2013 to April 2015 we conducted a randomized controlled trial with a parallel group design. Participants were randomly assigned to either an experimental group (perturbational treadmill training = PTT) or a control group (conventional treadmill training = CTT) by using a computer-generated block-randomization, stratified by Hoehn & Yahr stage[41] (H&Y 1-2 and H&Y 2.5-3). The random allocation sequence was generated by an independent person (SS) not involved in assessment or intervention, and group assignment was concealed during enrollment of participants at the hospital (University hospital Erlangen, Germany). The Ethics Committee of the University of Erlangen – Nuremberg (Germany) approved this research project and all participants gave written informed consent prior to intervention.

Recruitment of participants and screening for eligibility was performed at the University hospital Erlangen (Department Molecular Neurology, Erlangen). Participants fulfilling all of the following criteria were included in the study: 1) diagnosis of idiopathic Parkinson's disease, 2) Hoehn & Yahr (H&Y) stage 1-3, 3) Unified Parkinson's Disease Rating Scale[42,43] (UPDRS) subscore gait ≥ 1, and 4) able to walk independently without an assistive device. Patients were excluded if 1) they were diagnosed with any neurological disease other than Parkinson's disease, 2) they suffered from any severe cardiovascular or orthopedic condition that would impact performing the assessments and/or intervention, and 3) they were not able to follow instructions from the assessor and/or care provider due to cognitive impairment. All participants were informed that they will be assigned to one of two treatment groups but were not told whether they received the experimental or control treatment.

2.2 Intervention

Participants in the experimental group walked on a novel treadmill device (Zebris medical GmbH & h/p/cosmos medical GmbH), which applies additional perturbations during walking and thereby creates further challenges to postural control systems. For perturbational treadmill training (PTT), three pneumatic actuators below the treadmill (lifting capacity 8 cm; air pressure = 3.5 bar) constantly induced small three-dimensional tilting movements of the treadmill and thereby created an uneven surface while walking (Figure 1). The tilting platform can be switched on/off independent from the regular belt movement of the treadmill. The novel treadmill device is also equipped with handrails on the left and right side of the belt and with a suspension for a safety harness.

Participants in the control group performed conventional treadmill training (CTT), without additional perturbations applied. Control subjects walked on the same treadmill device as the experimental group but without additional perturbations (tilting platform switched off).

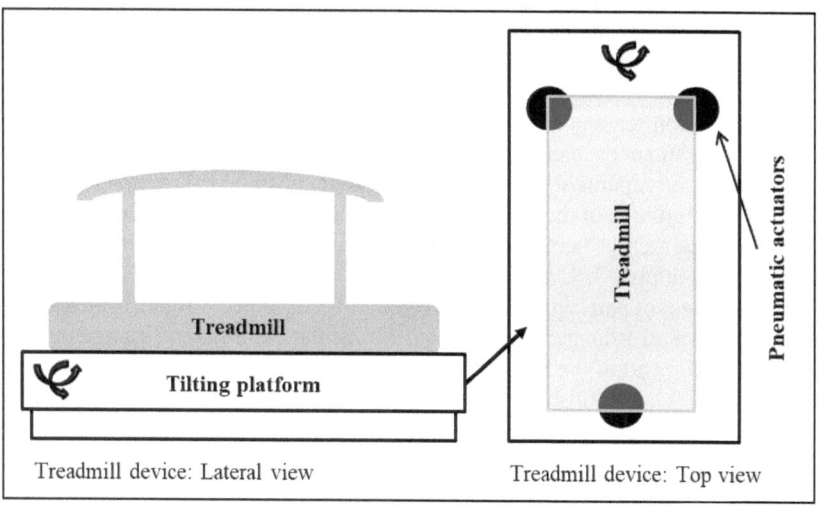

Figure 1:   Treadmill device

For both the experimental and control intervention the same standardized protocol was applied (Figure 2), which was designed based on a previous study [44] At first, all participants walked five minutes on the treadmill with their preferred speed to get familiar with the device; for PD patients in the experimental group the additional perturbations were switched on in the last minute of the familiarization period. Subsequently, all participants received a single session of 15 minutes treadmill training and based on their group assignment they walked with the perturbational stimulus (experimental) or without (control). Training was separated into three 5-minute-blocks with a rest period of three minutes (participants standing on the treadmill) between blocks. On the treadmill, patients walked with 70 % of their self-selected comfortable overground walking speed (10 Meter Walk Test) and were asked to walk without handrail support, if possible. For safety reasons, the care provider (SK) gave minimal instructions during the familiarization period on the treadmill, but no further recommendations regarding walking performance were provided.

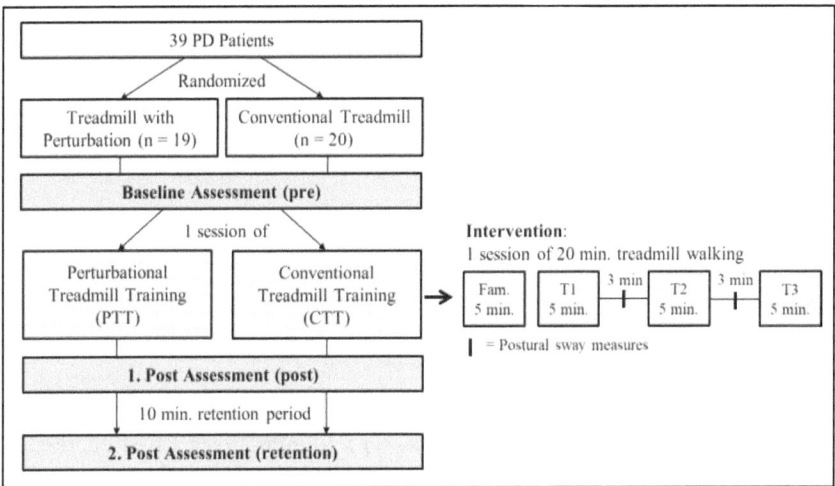

Figure 2:   Study protocol

2.3 Data Collection and Analysis

According to the study protocol (Figure 2) all data were collected at the same place (Institute of Sport Science and Sport, Erlangen, Germany) and at the same day as the intervention was performed, and by the same person who provided treadmill training (SK). All patients were assessed during their 'on' state of antiparkinson medication.

Primary outcome measures were self-selected comfortable overground walking speed and postural sway parameters (Center of pressure sway velocity [vCOP], - sway area [aCOP]). All primary outcome measures were assessed prior to (pre), immediately after (post) and 10 minutes after (retention) treadmill walking. In addition, postural sway parameters were measured between treadmill training, after the first training block (T1) and after the second training block (T2). Overground walking speed was assessed with 10 Meter Walk Test[45] and out of three attempts the average speed was calculated. Postural sway parameters were measured with a forceplate integrated in the treadmill (FDM-T, Zebris medical GmbH) during 30 seconds of quiet stance with eyes open. To avoid fatigue of multiple testing participants performed three attempts prior to intervention, two attempts at post and retention assessment, and one attempt between training blocks. For multiple attempts the average was calculated.[46]

Secondary outcome measures were spatiotemporal gait parameters assessed during treadmill walking without perturbations (e.g. stride length, step width, double limb support) on a forceplate (FDM-T, Zebris medical GmbH) for 60 seconds at the end of each training block and after the retention period. In addition, symmetry (Formula 1) and variability (Formula 2) of spatiotemporal gait parameters were calculated. Handrail support during treadmill walking was documented.

Formula (1):

Symmetry = $| \text{mean}_{left} - \text{mean}_{right} |$

Formula (2):

Variability = $\left(\dfrac{\text{standard deviation}}{\text{mean}} \right) * 100\ \%$

Statistical analysis was performed with IBM SPSS Statistics for Windows version 23.0 (IBM Corp. Released 2015; Armonk, NY). In order to get a first impression of the results and to choose the appropriate method for statistical analysis, a descriptive data analysis with various diagrams (e.g. growths rates of total sample, of treatment groups and individual growths rates) for every primary and secondary outcome measure was conducted.

In a second step, a two-level linear mixed model was developed to analyze growth rates over time (Level 1: within-individuals) and between-subjects effects (Level 2) of the main outcomes. The variables *time* (occasions of measurement: pre = 0, T1 = 1, T2 = 2, post = 3, retention = 4) and *group* (control = 0, experimental = 1) were included as covariates at Level 2. In order to be more flexible with varying occasions of measurement and individual variability a random intercept and random slope model was used. The assumed covariance matrix was diagonal for Level 1 and unstructured for Level 2. At first, changes over time within groups were investigated by entering the variable *time* as only covariate to the mixed model analysis of every primary and secondary outcome measure, and analyzing results separately for each group (split file by group). Afterwards, significant differences over time between groups were analyzed by adding the variables *time* and *group* as covariates to the model. In this part of the analysis main effects for *group* and *time*, as well as cross-level interactions (group x time) were analyzed.

As a last step of the statistical analysis *predictors* were integrated into the model, in order to explain differences in patients' growth rates (over time) in outcome measures. The following variables were chosen as potential *predictors* and were added as covariates separately to the existing model: falls rate, UPDRS, vCOP at baseline, and handrail usage. Predictors' main effect and cross-level interactions (time x predictor; group x time x predictor) were investigated. For better interpretation of the observed results, change scores (Formula 3) and standardized effect sizes were calculated (Formula 4). In addition, significant differences between groups in sample characteristics were analyzed with paired t-tests.

Formula (3):

$$\text{Change score} = \left(\frac{(\text{Mean}_{measurement\ occasion} - \text{Mean}_{baseline})}{\text{Mean baseline}} \right) \times 100\ \%$$

Formula (4):

$$\text{Effect size (Cohen's } d) = \left(\frac{\text{Estimate of effect}}{(\text{Standard Error}_{estimate\ of\ effect} \times \sqrt{\text{sample size}})} \right)$$

3   Results

3.1 Sample Charactersistics

Characteristics of 39 PD patients who were randomized into perturbational tread-mill training (n = 19) or conventional treadmill training (n = 20) are presented in Table 1. The average age of participants was 64.8 years in experimental group and 64.2 years in control group. People in both groups showed similar mean UPDRS scores (PTT = 16.7; CTT = 17.7) and the same amount of people (n = 8) had previous treadmill experience (ever walked on a treadmill). There were significantly more females in the perturbational treadmill group (PTT: n = 8; CTT: n = 2), compared to the control group. Frequency distribution of fall rates was different within groups but the number of fallers (PTT n = 12; CTT n = 10) and non-fallers (PTT n = 7; CTT n = 9) is comparable in experimental and control group.

Table 1:   Sample characteristics with mean SD or number of particpants (%)

	Experimental Group (PTT) n=19	Control Group (CTT) n=20	p-value[a]
Age (years)	64,8 ± 10,3	64,2 ± 8,5	.833
Gender (male/femal)*	11 / 8	18 / 2	.021 *
Height (cm)	173,9 ± 8,0	175,2 ± 13,7	.731
Weight (kg)	74,9 ± 13,0	83,2 ± 13,7	.060
UPDRS[b]	16,7 ± 5,5	17,7 ± 8,7	.662
Number of falls past 12 months[c] (percentage of participants)			.106
none	n=7 (36.8%)	n=9 (47.4%)	
one	n=3 (15.8%)	n=8 (42.1%)	
two	n=5 (26.3%)	n=0 (0%)	
three or more	n=4 (21.1%)	n=2 (10.6%)	
Treadmill experience[b] (percentage of participants)	n=8 (42.1%)	n=8 (40.0%)	1.0

[a] significant differences between groups calculated wth paired t-tests; [b] data from n=36; [c] data from n=38;
* significant at level $p \leq .05$

3.2 Gait and Postural Control

Results for primary outcome measures are presented in Table 2 and Table 3. Prior to treadmill intervention no significant differences between groups in primary outcome measures were observed. Participants in the perturbational treadmill group showed a significantly higher overground walking speed immediately after (post) and 10 minutes after (retention) intervention (p = .049; ES = +0.34), with a significant difference compared to the control group (p = .014; ES = +0.41) (Figure 3).

Center of pressure sway velocity decreased in both groups after retention below baseline values but without reaching statistical significance. In both groups center of pressure sway area increased over time, but only within the control group results were significant (p = .009; ES = +0.49) (Figure 3).

Table 2:   Primary outcome measures: Time effects within groups and group-by-time interaction effects (between groups) are reported with effect size (ES) and p-value.

Outcome measure	Time effects			
	within groups[a]		between groups[b]	
	ES	p-value	ES	p-value
Overground walking speed (m/s)				
experimental	+0.34	.049*		
			+0.41	.014*
control	-0.17	.440		
vCOP (mm/s)				
experimental	+0.14	.400		
			+0.17	.285
control	-0.14	.397		
aCOP (mm^2)				
experimental	+0.21	.197		
			-0.13	.416
control	+0.49	.009*		

[a] reference category: time=pre; [b] reference categories: time=pre, group=control
*significant at level p≤.05

Table 3: Primary outcome measures: Mean (SD) at baseline (pre) and mean change (SD) with change in % at T1, T2, post and retention.

	pre	T1		T2		post		retention	
	Mean (SD)	Mean change (SD)	%	Mean change (SD)	%	Mean change (SD)	%	Mean change (SD)	%
Overground walking speed (m/s)									
experimental	1.32 (0.19)	NA		NA		+0.03 (0.14)	+2.3%	+0.06 (0.13)	+4.7%
control	1.38 (0.20)	NA		NA		-0.05 (0.08)	-3.7%	-0.02 (0.10)	-1.7%
vCOP (mm/s)									
experimental	9.6 (5.66)	+0.34 (1.46)	+3.5%	+0.3 (1.47)	+3.1%	+0.81 (1.56)	+8.4%	-0.35 (1.51)	-3.6%
control	11.68 (5.99)	-0.15 (2.20)	-1.3%	+0.1 (1.64)	+0.9%	+0.04 (2.53)	+0.3%	-1.12 (2.70)	-9.6%
aCOP (mm^2)									
experimental	597.65 (363.88)	+164.74 (445.53)	+27.6%	+37.07 (555.67)	+6.2%	+187.73 (338.00)	+31.4%	+63.46 (265.27)	+10.6%
control	645.66 (440.08)	+64.02 (362.41)	+9.9%	+375.22 (505.23)	+58.1%	+239.5 (376.47)	+37.1%	+118.91 (346.53)	+20.6%

Measurement occasions

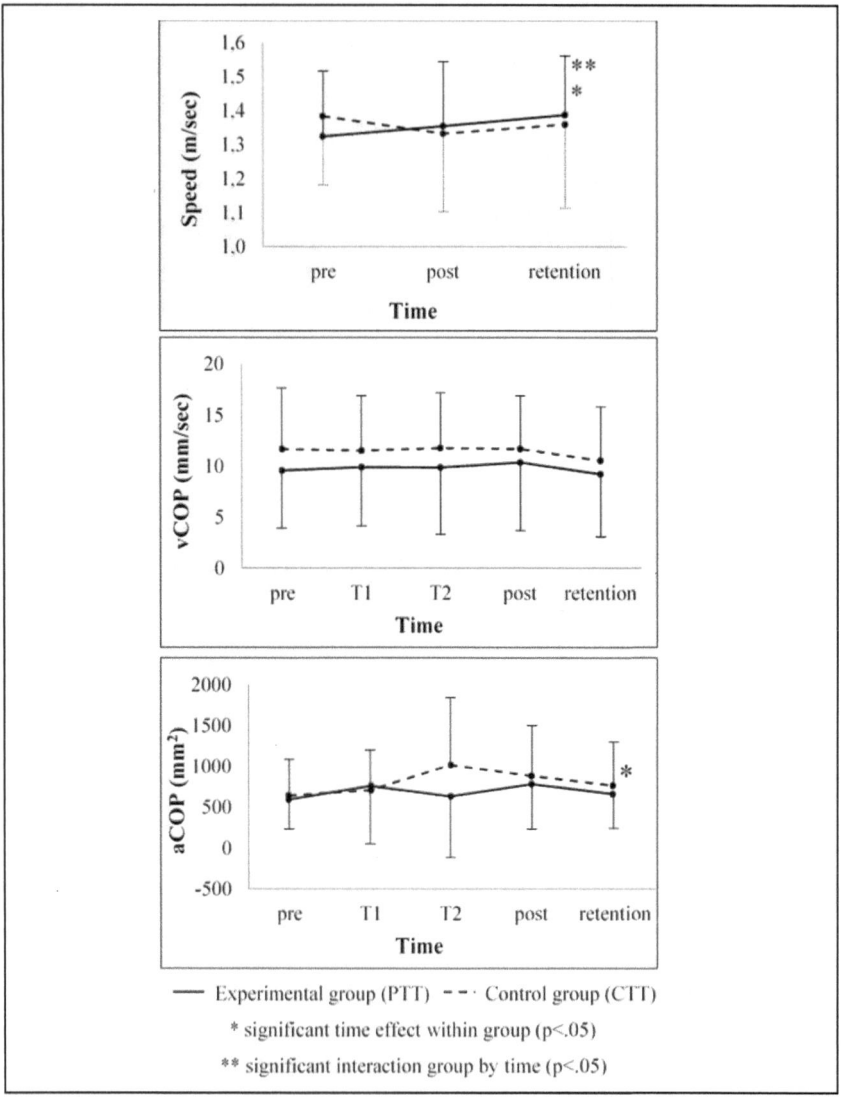

Figure 3:   Primary outcome measures

Analysis of spatiotemporal gait parameter during treadmill walking (Table 4 and Table 5) revealed a significant reduction in variability of stride length (p = .048; ES = -0.34), stride time (p = .052; ES = -0.33), double limb support (p = .005; ES = -0.48) and cadence (p = .048; ES = -0.34) for participants in the experimental group. Changes in gait variability over time did not significantly differ between groups. Step time symmetry during treadmill walking demonstrated a significant group by time interaction (p = .033; ES = -0.36), suggesting that participants in the control group decreased and the experimental group increased symmetry over time. None of the other spatiotemporal gait parameters showed significant changes over time within or between groups.

Additional results from the analysis of primary and secondary outcome measures are presented in Figure 4 and Table 6 and Table 7.

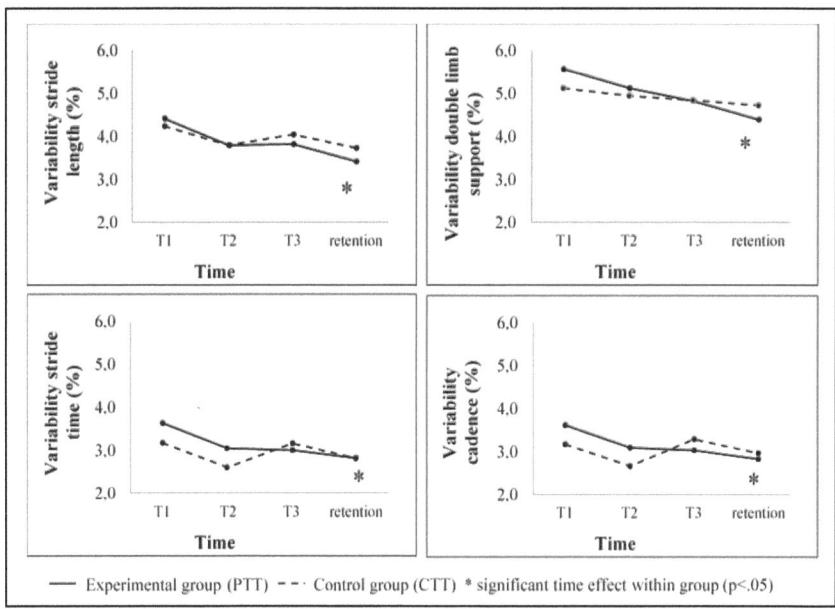

Figure 4:   Variability of spatiotemporal outcome measures

Table 4:   Secondary outcome measures: Mean (SD) at the beginning of the intervention (T1) and mean change (SD) with change in % at T2, post and retention.

	T1 Mean (SD)	T2 Mean change (SD)	%	post Mean change (SD)	%	retention Mean change (SD)	%
Stride length (cm)							
experimental	108.91 (16.26)	+1.21 (5.93)	+1.1%	+0.38 (5.24)	+0.3%	+1.08 (8.29)	+1.0%
control	110.70 (15.76)	-0.34 (5.60)	-0.3%	-0.34 (4.94)	+0.3%	-0.19 (5.04)	-0.2%
Step width (cm)							
experimental	10.12 (2.64)	-0.17 (1.40)	-1.7%	-0.06 (1.31)	-0.6%	-0.70 (1.42)	-6.9%
control	10.92 (3.08)	+0.50 (1.46)	+4.6%	+0.29 (1.21)	+2.7%	+0.23 (1.48)	+2.1%
Stride time (s)							
experimental	1.22 (0.16)	-0.01 (0.08)	+0.8%	+0.00 (0.07)	+0.0%	+0.01 (0.11)	+0.8%
control	1.15 (0.09)	+0.00 (0.07)	+0.0%	+0.00 (0.06)	+0.0%	+0.00 (0.06)	+0.0%
Double limb support (%)							
experimental	33.99 (3.49)	+0.00 (1.15)	+0.0%	+0.20 (1.31)	+0.6%	-0.03 (2.04)	-0.1%
control	35.09 (4.40)	+0.17 (0.97)	+0.5%	+0.14 (1.15)	+0.4%	+0.03 (1.03)	+0.1%
Cadence (steps/m)							
experimental	99.92 (12.83)	-1.20 (5.55)	-1.2%	-0.62 (4.76)	-0.6%	-1.33 (7.46)	-1.3%
control	104.66 (7.97)	+0.19 (5.12)	+0.2%	-0.56 (4.43)	-0.5%	-0.05 (4.71)	+0.0%
Variability stride length (%)							
experimental	4.33 (2.33)	-0.53 (1.53)	-12.2%	-0.60 (2.15)	-13.9%	-1.00 (1.49)	-23.1%
control	4.24 (2.95)	-0.44 (2.97)	-10.4%	-0.20 (1.64)	-4.7%	-0.51 (1.37)	-12%
Variability step width (%)							
experimental	18.39 (7.73)	+2.04 (5.14)	+11.1%	+1.84 (4.88)	+10.0%	-0.63 (6.55)	-3.4%
control	15.37 (7.06)	+1.92 (4.77)	+12.5%	+2.18 (6.93)	+14.2%	+1.64 (4.56)	+10.7%
Variability stride time (%)							
experimental	3.58 (1.81)	-0.52 (1.34)	-14.5%	+1.42 (1.72)	+39.7%	-0.81 (1.53)	-22.6%
control	3.18 (2.52)	-0.57 (2.49)	-17.9%	-0.01 (1.35)	-0.3%	-0.35 (1.17)	-11.0%
Variability double limb support (%)							
experimental	5.53 (2.03)	-0.40 (1.64)	-7.2%	-0.75 (1.43)	-13.6%	-1.17 (1.77)	-21.2%
control	5.13 (1.99)	-0.18 (2.39)	-3.5%	-0.28 (1.42)	-5.5%	-0.41 (1.42)	-8.0%
Variability cadence (%)							
experimental	3.56 (1.85)	-0.46 (1.31)	-12.9%	-0.58 (1.78)	-16.3%	-0.79 (1.50)	-22.2%
control	3.18 (2.56)	-0.50 (2.50)	-15.7%	+0.12 (1.07)	+3.8%	-0.21 (0.69)	-6.6%
Symmetry step length (cm)[a]							
experimental	2.84 (2.71)	+0.63 (1.77)	+22.2%	+1.09 (2.47)	+38.4%	+0.51 (1.51)	+18.0%
control	4.19 (3.27)	-0.17 (2.80)	-4.1%	-0.71 (2.57)	-16.9%	-0.48 (2.25)	-11.5%
Symmetry step time (ms)[a]							
experimental	24.20 (26.40)	-1.16 (12.65)	-4.8%	-1.64 (9.80)	-6.8%	-1.54 (13.79)	-6.4%
control	15.64 (11.20)	+1.03 (7.88)	+6.6%	+4.75 (9.83)	+30.4%	+5.23 (7.92)	+33.4%
Symmetry stance phase (%)[a]							
experimental	1.50 (1.43)	-0.09 (0.72)	-6.0%	-0.06 (0.68)	-4.0%	-0.27 (1.12)	-18.0%
control	0.94 (0.90)	+0.20 (0.70)	+21.3%	+0.24 (0.72)	+25.5%	+0.28 (0.67)	+29.8%

[a] difference between left and right leg (lower values indicate higher symmetry)

Table 5:   Secondary outcome measures: Time effects within groups and group-by-time interaction effects (between groups) are reported with effect size (ES) and p-value

| | Time effect | | | |
| | within groups[a] | | between groups[b] | |
	ES	p-value	ES	p-value
Stride length (cm)				
experimental	+0.01	.935		
			+0.02	.925
control	+0.00	.983		
Step width (cm)				
experimental	-0.11	.512		
			-0.23	.160
control	+0.09	.598		
Stride time (s)				
experimental	+0.01	.959		
			+0.01	.934
control	+0.00	.993		
Double limb support (%)				
experimental	+0.05	.743		
			+0.00	.981
control	-0.01	.973		
Cadence (steps/m)				
experimental	-0.07	.657		
			-0.02	.880
control	-0.06	.724		
Variability stride length (%)				
experimental	-0.34	.048*		
			-0.17	.292
control	-0.27	.117		
Variability step width (%)				
experimental	-0.11	.520		
			-0.23	.155
control	+0.11	.502		
Variability stride time (%)				
experimental	-0.33	.052*		
			-0.19	.232
control	-0.03	.870		
Variability double limb support (%)				
experimental	-0.48	.005*		
			-0.24	.148
control	-0.22	.180		
Variability cadence (%)				
experimental	-0.34	.048*		
			-0.17	.289
control	+0.01	.950		
Symmetry step length (cm)[c]				
experimental	+0.27	.112		
			+0.31	.059
control	-0.21	.206		
Symmetry step time (ms)[c]				
experimental	-0.11	.488		
			-0.36	.033*
control	+0.46	.010*		
Symmetry stance phase (%)[c]				
experimental	-0.12	.470		
			-0.29	.081
control	+0.24	.154		

[a] reference category: time=T1; [b] reference categories: time=T1, group=control
*significant at level p≤.05

Table 6: Primary and secondary outcome measures with mean±SD for all measurement occasions.

	pre	T1	T2	post	retention
	Mean ± SD	Mean ± SD	Mean ± SD	Mean ± SD	Mean ± SD
Overground walking speed (m/s)					
experimental	1,3 ± 0,2	NA	NA	1,4 ± 0,2	1,4 ± 0,2
control	1,4 ± 0,2	NA	NA	1,3 ± 0,2	1,4 ± 0,3
vCOP (mm/s)					
experimental	9,6 ± 5,7	9,9 ± 5,8	9,9 ± 6,6	10,4 ± 6,7	9,3 ± 6,1
control	11,7 ± 6,0	11,5 ± 5,4	11,8 ± 5,4	11,7 ± 5,2	10,6 ± 5,3
aCOP (mm^2)					
experimental	597,7 ± 363,9	762,4 ± 709,9	634,7 ± 748,7	785,4 ± 550,0	661,1 ± 417,0
control	645,7 ± 440,1	709,7 ± 496,0	1020,9 ± 827,1	885,2 ± 617,9	764,6 ± 538,1
Stride length (cm)					
experimental	NA	108,9 ± 16,3	110,1 ± 15,3	109,3 ± 14,2	110,0 ± 15,9
control	NA	110,7 ± 15,8	110,1 ± 15,8	111,0 ± 15,6	110,5 ± 15,4
Step width (cm)					
experimental	NA	10,1 ± 2,6	9,9 ± 2,6	10,1 ± 2,4	9,4 ± 2,3
control	NA	10,9 ± 3,1	11,4 ± 3,1	11,2 ± 3,3	11,2 ± 3,0
Stride time (s)					
experimental	NA	1,2 ± 0,2	1,2 ± 0,2	1,2 ± 0,2	1,2 ± 0,2
control	NA	1,2 ± 0,1	1,2 ± 0,1	1,2 ± 0,1	1,2 ± 0,1
Double limb support (%)					
experimental	NA	34,0 ± 3,5	34,0 ± 3,3	34,2 ± 3,5	34,0 ± 4,0
control	NA	35,1 ± 4,4	35,1 ± 4,2	35,2 ± 4,4	35,1 ± 4,0
Cadence (steps/m)					
experimental	NA	99,9 ± 12,8	98,7 ± 12,4	99,3 ± 11,8	98,6 ± 11,6
control	NA	104,7 ± 8,0	105,4 ± 7,5	104,1 ± 5,7	104,6 ± 6,3

Measurement occasions

[a] difference between left and right leg (lower values indicate higher symmetry)

Table 6: Continued

	Measurement occasions									
	pre	T1		T2		post		retention	
	Mean ± SD	Mean ± SD		Mean ± SD		Mean ± SD		Mean ± SD	
Variability stride length (%)										
experimental	NA	4,3	± 2,3	3,8	± 1,7	3,8	± 2,2	3,4	± 1,7
control	NA	4,2	± 3,0	3,8	± 1,7	4,1	± 1,7	3,7	± 1,9
Variability step width (%)										
experimental	NA	18,4	± 7,7	20,4	± 6,7	20,2	± 5,9	17,6	± 5,6
control	NA	15,4	± 7,1	17,3	± 6,3	17,6	± 8,0	17,0	± 7,7
Variability stride time (%)										
experimental	NA	3,6	± 1,8	3,1	± 1,6	3,0	± 1,9	2,8	± 1,6
control	NA	3,2	± 2,5	2,6	± 1,1	3,2	± 1,6	2,8	± 1,6
Variability double limb supp										
experimental	NA	5,5	± 2,0	5,1	± 1,7	4,8	± 1,7	4,4	± 1,1
control	NA	5,1	± 2,0	5,0	± 1,5	4,8	± 1,3	4,7	± 1,0
Variability cadence (%)										
experimental	NA	3,6	± 1,9	3,1	± 1,6	3,1	± 2,0	2,8	± 1,5
control	NA	3,2	± 2,6	2,7	± 1,1	3,3	± 2,2	3,0	± 2,3
Symmetry step length (cm)[a]										
experimental	NA	2,8	± 2,7	3,5	± 3,3	3,9	± 4,1	3,4	± 2,5
control	NA	4,2	± 3,3	4,2	± 2,7	3,5	± 2,3	3,7	± 2,8
Symmetry step time (ms)[a]										
experimental	NA	24,2	± 26,4	23,0	± 23,4	22,6	± 23,4	22,7	± 21,9
control	NA	16,4	± 11,2	17,5	± 11,0	20,8	± 12,6	21,7	± 13,3
Symmetry stance phase (%)[a]										
experimental	NA	1,5	± 1,4	1,4	± 1,4	1,4	± 1,2	1,2	± 1,1
control	NA	0,9	± 0,9	1,2	± 0,8	1,2	± 1,1	1,3	± 0,9

[a] difference between left and right leg (lower values indicate higher symmetry)

Table 7: Primary and secondary outcome measures: Time effects within groups and between groups reported with estimate of effect, standard error (SE) and p-value

| | Time effects | | | | | |
| | within groups[a] | | | between groups[b] | | |
	Estimate	SE	p-value	Estimate	SE	p-value
Overground walking speed (m/s)						
experimental	0,03	0,01	.049*			
				0,05	0,02	.014*
control	-0,01	0,01	.440			
vCOP (mm/s)						
experimental	0,08	0,10	.400			
				0,19	0,17	.285
control	-0,14	0,15	.387			
aCOP (mm^2)						
experimental	20,32	15,15	.197			
				-20,19	24,52	.416
control	67,51	22,05	.009*			
Stride length (cm)						
experimental	0,04	0,51	.935			
				0,06	0,65	.925
control	0,01	0,36	.983			
Step width (cm)						
experimental	-0,07	0,10	.512			
				-0,21	0,15	.160
control	0,05	0,10	.598			
Stride time (s)						
experimental	0,00	0,01	.959			
				0,00	0,01	.934
control	0,00	0,00	.993			
Double limb support (%)						
experimental	0,04	0,13	.743			
				0,00	0,16	.981
control	0,00	0,07	.973			
Cadence (steps/m)						
experimental	-0,21	0,46	.657			
				-0,09	0,59	.880
control	-0,13	0,37	.724			

[a] reference category: time=pre/T1; [b] reference categories: time=pre/T1, group=control
*significant at level p≤.05

Table 7:   Continued

	Time effects					
	within groups[a]			between groups[b]		
	Estimate	SE	p-value	Estimate	SE	p-value
Variability stride length (%)						
experimental	-0,26	0,12	.048*			
				-0,17	0,16	.292
control	-0,18	0,10	.117			
Variability step width (%)						
experimental	-0,30	0,45	.520			
				-0,82	0,57	.155
control	0,28	0,41	.502			
Variability stride time (%)						
experimental	-0,24	0,12	.052*			
				-0,17	0,14	.232
control	-0,03	0,17	.870			
Variability double limb support (%)						
experimental	-0,37	0,13	.005*			
				-0,25	0,17	.148
control	-0,13	0,09	.180			
Variability cadence (%)						
experimental	-0,24	0,11	.048*			
				-0,25	0,23	.289
control	0,01	0,20	.950			
Symmetry step length (cm)						
experimental	0,35	0,21	.112			
				0,41	0,21	.059
control	-0,23	0,17	.206			
Symmetry step time (ms)						
experimental	-0,65	0,92	.488			
				-2,53	1,14	.033*
control	1,75	0,61	.010*			
Symmetry stance phase (%)						
experimental	-0,06	0,07	.470			
				-0,17	0,10	.081
control	0,07	0,05	.154			

[a] reference category: time=pre/T1; [b] reference categories: time=pre/T1, group=control
*significant at level p≤.05

3.3 Predictors

In the experimental group 15 % and in the control group 21 % of participants were able to walk without holding on the handrails during the whole treadmill training. The other participants made use of handrails either partially during training (PTT: 45 %; CTT: 42 %) or throughout the whole session (PTT: 40 %; CTT: 37 %). Handrail support affected growth rates during treadmill training for people in the experimental group but not in the control group (Figure 5). If PD patients trained with the perturbational stimulus, walking without support by handrails predicted a reduced variability of cadence (p = .002; ES = -0.52) and a higher step time symmetry (p = .029; ES = -0.36) over time compared to walking with handrail support.

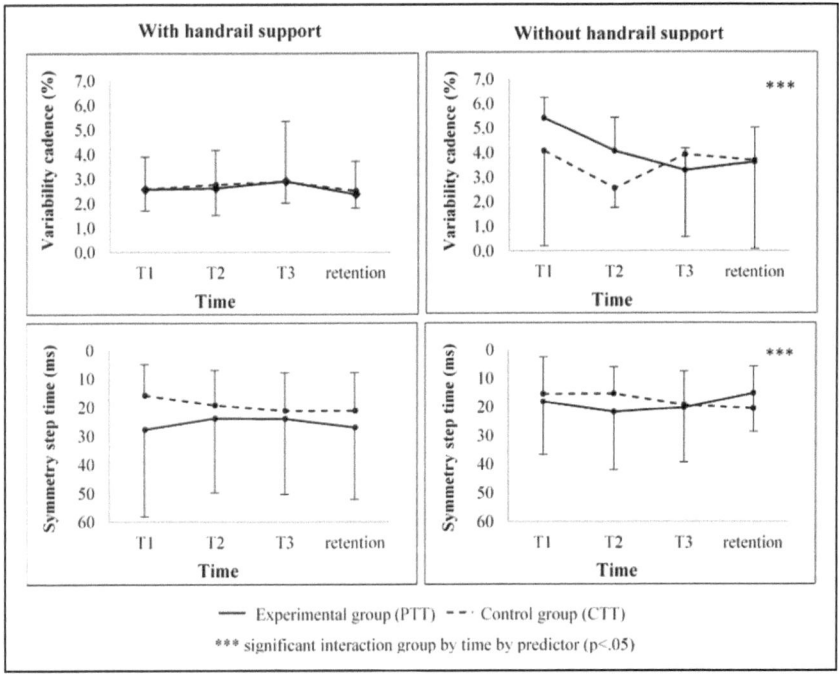

Figure 5:   Predictor handrail support

Including patients' impairment and disease severity into the analysis revealed that participants with higher fall rates showed a larger increase in overground walking speed (p = .016; ES = +0.40) and stance phase symmetry (p = .011; ES =

-0.42) over time, if they trained with the perturbational stimulus (Figure 6). Integrating patients' UPDRS score supported these results, indicating that a higher UPDRS also predicted a larger increase in overground walking speed (p = .042; ES = +0.34) and in stance phase symmetry (p = .045; ES = -0.33) for people in the experimental group. Center of pressure sway velocity at baseline did not show significant predictions for growth rates in primary or secondary outcomes.

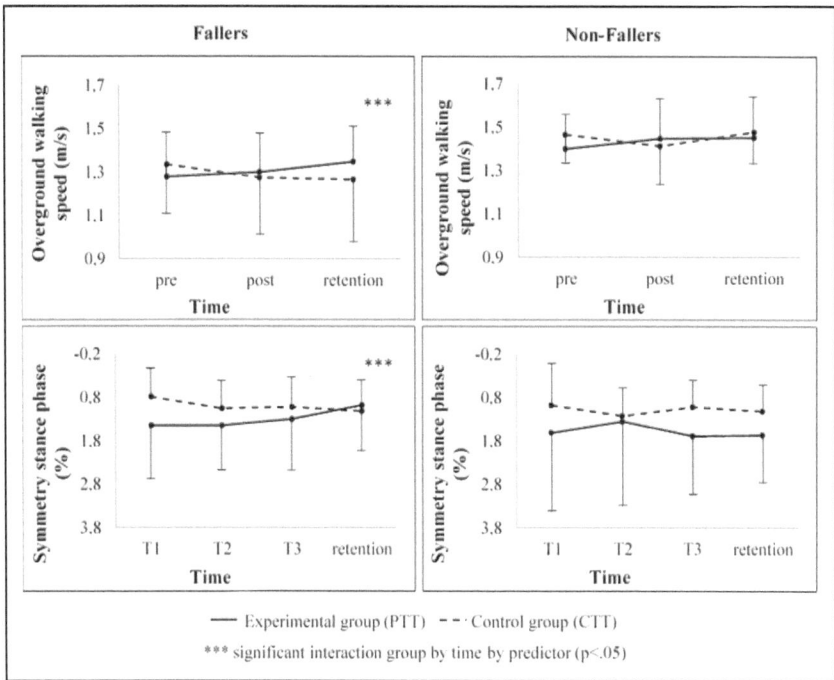

Figure 6:   Predictor fall rate

Effects of all predictors (fall rate, UPDRS, vCOP baseline, handrail support) on growth rates of primary and secondary outcomes are presented in Table 8.

Table 8:   Effects of predictors on growth rates of primary and secondary outcomes. Interaction effects reported with estimate of effect, standard error (SE), p-value

| | Interaction effects | | | | | |
| | time-by-predictor[a] | | | time-by-predictor-by-group[a,b] | | |
	Estimate	SE	p-value	Estimate	SE	p-value
Fall rate						
OWS (m/s)	0,01	0,01	.388	0,02	0,01	.016*
vCOP (mm/s)	0,002	0,08	.956	0,07	0,09	.445
aCOP	7,67	10,24	.459	-5,49	10,50	.604
Stride length (cm)	-0,13	0,31	.680	0,15	0,31	.640
Step width (cm)	-0,05	0,07	.503	-0,08	0,07	.277
Stride time (s)	0,00	0,00	.973	0,00	0,00	.568
Double limb support (%)	0,05	0,07	.481	-0,02	0,08	.755
Cadence (steps/m)	0,11	0,27	.697	-0,07	0,27	.799
Variability stride length (%)	-0,09	0,07	.245	-0,08	0,07	.231
Variability step width (%)	-0,26	0,27	.335	-0,29	0,27	.280
Variability stride time (%)	-0,03	0,07	.643	-0,05	0,06	.447
Variability double limb support (%)	-0,06	0,08	.442	-0,07	0,08	.353
Variability cadence (%)	-0,05	0,11	.678	-0,09	0,11	.433
Symmetry step length (cm)	0,02	0,11	.846	0,03	0,10	.799
Symmetry step time (ms)	-0,42	0,52	.421	-0,64	0,51	.215
Symmetry stance phase (%)	-0,05	0,04	.301	-0,10	0,04	.011*
UPDRS						
OWS (m/s)	0,00	0,00	.701	0,00	0,00	.042*
vCOP	-0,04	0,01	.003*	0,01	0,01	.446
aCOP	0,04	1,93	.982	-1,39	1,56	.381
Stride length (cm)	-0,05	0,05	.263	-0,03	0,04	.427
Step width (cm)	0,01	0,01	.466	-0,01	0,01	.277
Stride time (s)	0,00	0,00	.230	0,00	0,00	.400
Double limb support (%)	0,00	0,01	.757	0,00	0,01	.929
Cadence (steps/m)	0,04	0,04	.333	0,03	0,03	.394
Variability stride length (%)	0,00	0,01	.988	-0,01	0,01	.135
Variability step width (%)	0,02	0,04	.621	-0,02	0,03	.497
Variability stride time (%)	0,00	0,01	.761	-0,01	0,01	.295
Variability double limb support (%)	0,00	0,01	.914	-0,01	0,01	.207
Variability cadence (%)	0,01	0,02	.686	-0,01	0,02	.360
Symmetry step length (cm)[c]	-0,02	0,02	.127	0,01	0,01	.360
Symmetry step time (ms)[c]	0,00	0,00	.443	-0,11	0,07	.143
Symmetry stance phase (%)[c]	0,00	0,01	.640	-0,01	0,01	.045*

[a] reference categories: time=pre/T1, predictor=lowest value;
[b] reference categories: time=pre/T1, predictor=lowest value, group=control;
[c] lower values/scores indicate better performance;
*significant at level p≤.05

Table 8: Continued

	Interaction effects					
	time-by-predictor[a]			time-by-predictor-by-group[a,b]		
	Estimate	SE	p-value	Estimate	SE	p-value
vCOP Baseline						
OWS (m/s)	0,00	0,00	.033*	0,00	0,00	.089
Stride length (cm)	-0,03	0,06	.564	-0,01	0,05	.901
Step width (cm)	0,00	0,01	.836	-0,01	0,01	.291
Stride time (s)	0,00	0,00	.579	0,00	0,00	.962
Double limb support (%)	0,00	0,01	.873	0,01	0,01	.515
Cadence (steps/m)	0,02	0,05	.730	0,00	0,05	.944
Variability stride length (%)	0,02	0,01	.247	0,00	0,01	.758
Variability step width (%)	0,02	0,05	.714	-0,01	0,05	.790
Variability stride time (%)	0,02	0,01	.139	0,00	0,01	.890
Variability double limb support (%)	0,01	0,01	.373	-0,01	0,01	.260
Variability cadence (%)	0,01	0,02	.733	-0,01	0,02	.654
Symmetry step length (cm)	-0,04	0,02	.018*	0,01	0,02	.634
Symmetry step time (ms)	0,12	0,10	.261	-0,16	0,09	.088
Symmetry stance phase (%)	0,01	0,01	.135	-0,01	0,01	.388
Handrailusage						
OWS (m/s)	0,00	0,00	.475	0,01	0,00	.131
vCOP	0,05	0,04	.243	0,03	0,04	.365
aCOP	-8,55	5,33	.117	-6,40	4,80	.191
Stride length (cm)	0,23	0,14	.113	0,13	0,13	.320
Step width (cm)	0,02	0,03	.575	0,00	0,03	.870
Stride time (s)	0,00	0,00	.130	0,00	0,00	.597
Double limb support (%)	-0,04	0,04	.264	-0,03	0,03	.327
Cadence (steps/m)	-0,20	0,13	.135	-0,08	0,11	.496
Variability stride length (%)	-0,03	0,03	.384	-0,03	0,03	.352
Variability step width (%)	0,22	0,13	.088	-0,14	0,11	.228
Variability stride time (%)	-0,04	0,03	.220	-0,04	0,03	.116
Variability double limb support (%)	-0,01	0,04	.760	-0,03	0,03	.277
Variability cadence (%)	-0,02	0,05	.749	-0,07	0,02	.002*
Symmetry step length (cm)	0,03	0,05	.595	0,06	0,04	.196
Symmetry step time (ms)	-0,22	0,27	.423	-0,50	0,22	.029*
Symmetry stance phase (%)	-0,01	0,02	.730	-0,02	0,02	.329

[a] reference categories: time=pre/T1, predictor=lowest value;
[b] reference categories: time=pre/T1, predictor=lowest value, group=control;
[c] lower values/scores indicate better performance; [d] with handrail support=0, without handrail support=1
*significant at level p≤.05

4 Discussion

This study investigated acute effects in gait and postural control in people with PD after a single session of perturbational treadmill training applying additional postural challenges during walking. Treadmill training with perturbations significantly increased overground walking speed after intervention, compared to conventional treadmill training. Measures of postural control revealed no significant changes over time between groups. Only the experimental group showed a significantly reduced gait variability during and after intervention. Further, walking without handrail support during perturbations predicted significantly larger improvements in step time symmetry and variability of cadence. More disabled PD patients seemed to benefit most from perturbational treadmill training.

Participants in the experimental group walked significantly faster over ground immediately after and 10 minutes after treadmill intervention. Previous research about sensorimotor adaptation might provide some explanations for these findings. The definition of 'motor adaptation' by Martin et al.47 suggested that people who adapted to a new motor behavior also have to de-adapt in order to achieve their prior behavior. Participants in the experimental group adapted their walking performance to perturbations by improving their gait variability and gait symmetry during treadmill walking which suggests an increased gait stability. Although perturbations were not present during overground walking, PD patients might not have been able to directly de-adapt after treadmill performance and used the more stable gait also overground which could have enabled them to walk faster. Other mechanisms which might explain the observed after-effects are feedforward adjustments and anticipatory control. Lam et al.48 showed that people adapted to dynamic perturbations while walking by using not only feedback but also feedforward control. When perturbations were removed, people still anticipated them and used their newly acquired adaptive strategies. Interestingly, participants in the present study showed adaptations in walking overground which might suggest that they transferred their motor behavior from treadmill walking. Reisman et al.49 also investigated acute effects of a type of perturbational treadmill training in stroke patients which transferred treadmill effects to overground walking, while healthy controls did not. The authors argued that this was due to difficulties with 'switching' environments for stroke survivors, and adaptation to different contexts may also play a role in individuals with PD.

To the best of our knowledge this was the first study investigating the effects of such a type of perturbational treadmill training in people with PD. Thus, comparing our findings with previous research is limited. Nevertheless, a few trials[16,15,50] examined acute adaptations after conventional treadmill training in PD which is comparable to our control intervention. Two of these studies[15,16] reported that patients significantly increased in overground walking speed and one showed improved gait variability[50] after intervention, while control subjects in the present study did not. It is important to note that participants in these studies were trained with the same speed[16,50] (or even higher)[15] on the treadmill as they walked overground, and they walked with hands on handrails. Since PD patients in our trial also walked without handrail support and trained only with 70 % of their overground walking speed, this might explain the different findings for conventional treadmill training.

We also aimed for identifying predictive variables which might explain differences in adaptations across participants. The role of handrails in treadmill training previously has been discussed[51] and pointed out as being important for future research[15]. Based on research with wheeled walkers[50,52], Bello and colleagues[51] suggested that handrail support has less impact on gait effects. However, our analysis revealed that walking without handrail support during perturbations led to significantly larger improvement in parameters indicating more gait stability (variability cadence, symmetry step time). Bastian[53] described motor adaptations as a 'trial-error-process', while errors during motor performance facilitated adaptation. People walking without handrail support during perturbations had no external support and needed to compensate perturbations solely by adapting their walking performance. This could have produced more errors in motor behavior, and thereby improved walking performance over time. Further, we showed that higher impairments of patients predicted significantly larger improvements in gait performance (overground walking speed, symmetry stance phase) when walking with the perturbational stimulus. This was supported by two predictors, fall status and UPDRS. These specific benefits for PD patients in advanced stages also have been reported for conventional treadmill training[16]. These results support the idea that adaptation seems to be largely intact in people with degenerative basal ganglia damage[54–56]. Nevertheless, one could hypothesize that more disabled PD patients, with higher cognitive impairments, have more difficulties with switching environments and contexts,[57,58] and thus study adaptation processes over a longer period of time.

The results of this study have to be interpreted with caution as there are several limitations. Quality of postural sway measures could have been improved by conducting three trials at every measurement occasion and performing quiet stance with eyes closed[46]. Measurement of spatiotemporal gait parameter during overground walking would have increased the meaningfulness of the observed changes in gait. Moreover, assessments and intervention were provided by the same person (SK) which was not blinded to group allocation. Although the sample size was relatively high compared to previous studies[14,15,16], high standard deviations in the results indicated large variations between participants. Finally, the allocation of males and females to treatment groups was unbalanced.

One of the main goals in rehabilitation is motor learning, which requires long-term exercise. Nevertheless, it is very important to investigate acute adaptations to new therapeutic techniques since motor adaptation is a prerequisite for motor learning[53]. In this study PD patients showed adaptations in gait after a single session of perturbational treadmill training. Future research needs to examine whether regular training with the novel treadmill device would lead to long-term changes in gait performance. Our findings indicate that the novel treadmill training is feasible for mild to moderately affected PD patients and thus would be a save technique in gait rehabilitation. An important next step would be to prove feasibility and effectiveness of the novel intervention in more severely impaired patients (H&Y $\geq$ 3) as their increased risk of falling[59] requires effective rehabilitative strategies. Moreover, this treadmill training with additional postural challenges might be also applicable for rehabilitation in other populations with gait and balance impairments.

5 Clinical Message

- Treadmill training with perturbations (creating an uneven surface) is feasible for mildly to moderately affected PD patients

- One session of perturbational treadmill training showed short-term improvements in overground walking speed and gait variability

- This novel technique might be also beneficial to other populations with gait and balance impairments

References

1. Wirdefeldt K, Adami H, Cole P, Trichopoulos D and Mandel J. Epidemiology and etiology of Parkinson's disease: a review of the evidence. Eur J Epidemiol 2011; 26 Suppl 1: S1-58.

2. Alves G, Forsaa EB, Pedersen KF, Dreetz Gjerstad M and Larsen JP. Epidemiology of Parkinson's disease. J Neurol 2008; 255 Suppl 5: 18–32.

3. Lees AJ, Hardy J and Revesz T. Parkinson's disease. Lancet 2009; 373: 2055–2066.

4. Kim SD, Allen NE, Canning CG and Fung, Victor S C. Postural instability in patients with Parkinson's disease. Epidemiology, pathophysiology and management. CNS Drugs 2013; 27: 97–112.

5. Soh S, Morris ME and McGinley JL. Determinants of health-related quality of life in Parkinson's disease: a systematic review. Parkinsonism Relat Disord 2011; 17: 1–9.

6. do Espirito Santo, C C, Swarowsky A, Recchia TL, Lopes, A P F and Ilha J. Is body weight-support treadmill training effective in increasing muscle trophism after traumatic spinal cord injury? A systematic review. Spinal Cord 2014.

7. English AW, Wilhelm JC and Sabatier MJ. Enhancing recovery from peripheral nerve injury using treadmill training. Ann Anat 2011; 193: 354–361.

8. Hicks AL and Ginis, Kathleen A Martin. Treadmill training after spinal cord injury: it's not just about the walking. J Rehabil Res Dev 2008; 45: 241–248.

9. Mehrholz J, Pohl M and Elsner B. Treadmill training and body weight support for walking after stroke. Cochrane Database Syst Rev 2014; 1: CD002840.

10. Molina-Rueda F, Aguila-Maturana AM, Molina-Rueda MJ and Miangolarra-Page JC. Treadmill training with or without partial body weight support in children with cerebral palsy: systematic review and meta-analysis. Rev Neurol 2010; 51: 135–145.

11. Schwartz I and Meiner Z. The influence of locomotor treatment using robotic body-weight-supported treadmill training on rehabilitation outcome of patients suffering from neurological disorders. Harefuah 2013; 152: 166-71, 182, 181.

12. Swinnen E, Beckwee D, Pinte D, Meeusen R, Baeyens J and Kerckhofs E. Treadmill training in multiple sclerosis: can body weight support or robot assistance provide added value? A systematic review. Mult Scler Int 2012; 2012: 240274.

13. Mehrholz J, Friis R, Kugler J, Twork S, Storch A and Pohl M. Treadmill training for patients with Parkinson's disease. Cochrane Database Syst Rev 2010: CD007830.

14. Miyai I, Fujimoto Y, Ueda Y, et al. Treadmill training with body weight support: its effect on Parkinson's disease. Arch Phys Med Rehabil 2000; 81: 849–852.

15. Pohl M, Rockstroh G, Ruckriem S, Mrass G and Mehrholz J. Immediate effects of speed-dependent treadmill training on gait parameters in early Parkinson's disease. Arch Phys Med Rehabil 2003; 84: 1760–1766.

16. Bello O, Sanchez JA and Fernandez-del-Olmo M. Treadmill walking in Parkinson's disease patients: adaptation and generalization effect. Mov. Disord. 2008; 23: 1243–1249.

17. Cakit BD, Saracoglu M, Genc H, Erdem HR and Inan L. The effects of incremental speed-dependent treadmill training on postural instability and fear of falling in Parkinson's disease. Clin Rehabil 2007; 21: 698–705.

18. Miyai I, Fujimoto Y, Yamamoto H, et al. Long-term effect of body weight-supported treadmill training in Parkinson's disease: a randomized controlled trial. Arch Phys Med Rehabil 2002; 83: 1370–1373.

19. Fisher BE, Wu AD, Salem GJ, et al. The effect of exercise training in improving motor performance and corticomotor excitability in people with early Parkinson's disease. Arch Phys Med Rehabil 2008; 89: 1221–1229.

20. Choi JT, Vining, Eileen P G, Reisman DS and Bastian AJ. Walking flexibility after hemispherectomy: split-belt treadmill adaptation and feedback control. Brain 2009; 132: 722–733.

21. Reisman DS, Wityk R, Silver K and Bastian AJ. Locomotor adaptation on a split-belt treadmill can improve walking symmetry post-stroke. Brain 2007; 130: 1861–1872.

22. Blanchette A, Lambert S, Richards CL and Bouyer LJ. Walking while resisting a perturbation: Effects on ankle dorsiflexor activation during swing and potential for rehabilitation. Gait Posture 2011; 34: 358–363.

23. IJmker T, Lamoth CJ, Houdijk H, van der Woude, Lucas H V and Beek PJ. Postural threat during walking: effects on energy cost and accompanying gait changes. J Neuroeng Rehabil 2014; 11: 71.

24. Hak L, Houdijk H, Steenbrink F, et al. Stepping strategies for regulating gait adaptability and stability. J Biomech 2013; 46: 905–911.

25. Parijat P, Lockhart TE and Liu J. Effects of perturbation-based slip training using a virtual reality environment on slip-induced falls. Ann Biomed Eng 2015; 43: 958–967.

26. Beurskens R, Wilken JM and Dingwell JB. Dynamic stability of individuals with transtibial amputation walking in destabilizing environments. J Biomech 2014; 47: 1675–1681.

27. Hof AL and Duysens J. Responses of human hip abductor muscles to lateral balance perturbations during walking. Exp Brain Res 2013; 230: 301–310.

28. Peterson MJ, Jongprasithporn M and Carey SL. Evaluation of Fall Recovery and Gait Adaptation to Medial and Lateral Gait Perturbations. Biomed Sci Instrum 2015; 51: 198–205.

29. Hnat SK and van den Bogert, Antonie J. Inertial compensation for belt acceleration in an instrumented treadmill. J Biomech 2014; 47: 3758–3761.

30. Ilmane N, Croteau S and Duclos C. Quantifying dynamic and postural balance difficulty during gait perturbations using stabilizing/destabilizing forces. J Biomech 2015; 48: 441–448.

31. Krasovsky T, Banina MC, Hacmon R, Feldman AG, Lamontagne A and Levin MF. Stability of gait and interlimb coordination in older adults. J Neurophysiol 2012; 107: 2560–2569.

32. Liu J and Kim S. Effect of walking surface perturbation training on slip propensity and local dynamic stability. Work 2012; 41 Suppl 1: 3352–3354.

33. Lurie JD, Zagaria AB, Pidgeon DM, Forman JL and Spratt KF. Pilot comparative effectiveness study of surface perturbation treadmill training to prevent falls in older adults. BMC Geriatr 2013; 13: 49.

34. Moore JK, Hnat SK and van den Bogert, Antonie J. An elaborate data set on human gait and the effect of mechanical perturbations. PeerJ 2015; 3: e918.

35. Obuchi S, Kojima M, Shiba Y, Shimada H and Suzuki T. A randomized controlled trial of a treadmill training with the perturbation to improve the balance performance in the community dwelling elderly subjects. Nihon Ronen Igakkai Zasshi 2004; 41: 321–327.

36. Sessoms PH, Wyatt M, Grabiner M, et al. Method for evoking a trip-like response using a treadmill-based perturbation during locomotion. J Biomech 2014; 47: 277–280.

37. Shapiro A and Melzer I. Balance perturbation system to improve balance compensatory responses during walking in old persons. J Neuroeng Rehabil 2010; 7: 32.

38. Shimada H, Obuchi S, Furuna T and Suzuki T. New intervention program for preventing falls among frail elderly people: the effects of perturbed walking exercise using a bilateral separated treadmill. Am J Phys Med Rehabil 2004; 83: 493–499.

39. Yang F, Bhatt T and Pai Y. Generalization of treadmill-slip training to prevent a fall following a sudden (novel) slip in over-ground walking. J Biomech 2013; 46: 63–69.

40. Allen NE, Sherrington C, Paul SS and Canning CG. Balance and falls in Parkinson's disease: a meta-analysis of the effect of exercise and motor training. Mov. Disord. 2011; 26: 1605–1615.

41. Hoehn MM and Yahr MD. Parkinsonism: onset, progression and mortality. Neurology 1967; 17: 427–442.

42. Fahn S and Elton RL. Unified Parkinon's disease rating scale. In: Fahn S, Goldstein M, Marsden D and Calne DB (eds) Recent developments in Parkinson's disease. New Yersey: MacMillan, 1987, pp. 153–163.

43. Ramaker C, Marinus J, Stiggelbout AM and Van Hilten, Bob Johannes. Systematic evaluation of rating scales for impairment and disability in Parkinson's disease. Mov. Disord. 2002; 17: 867–876.

44. Bello O, Sanchez JA and Fernandez-del-Olmo M. Treadmill walking in Parkinson's disease patients: adaptation and generalization effect. Mov. Disord. 2008; 23: 1243–1249.

45. Bohannon RW, Andrews AW and Thomas MW. Walking speed: reference values and correlates for older adults. J Orthop Sports Phys Ther 1996; 24: 86–90.

46. Ruhe A, Fejer R and Walker B. The test-retest reliability of centre of pressure measures in bipedal static task conditions--a systematic review of the literature. Gait Posture 2010; 32: 436–445.

47. Martin TA, Keating JG, Goodkin HP, Bastian AJ and Thach WT. Throwing while looking through prisms. II. Specificity and storage of multiple gaze-throw calibrations. Brain 1996; 119 (Pt 4): 1199–1211.

48. Lam T, Anderschitz M and Dietz V. Contribution of feedback and feedforward strategies to locomotor adaptations. J Neurophysiol 2006; 95: 766–773.

49. Reisman DS, Wityk R, Silver K and Bastian AJ. Split-belt treadmill adaptation transfers to overground walking in persons poststroke. Neurorehabil Neural Repair 2009; 23: 735–744.

50. Frenkel-Toledo S, Giladi N, Peretz C, Herman T, Gruendlinger L and Hausdorff JM. Treadmill walking as an external pacemaker to improve gait rhythm and stability in Parkinson's disease. Mov. Disord. 2005; 20: 1109–1114.

51. Bello O and Fernandez-del-Olmo M. How does the treadmill affect gait in Parkinson's disease? Curr Aging Sci 2012; 5: 28–34.

52. Cubo E, Moore CG, Leurgans S and Goetz CG. Wheeled and standard walkers in Parkinson's disease patients with gait freezing. Parkinsonism Relat Disord 2003; 10: 9–14.

53. Bastian AJ. Understanding sensorimotor adaptation and learning for rehabilitation. Curr Opin Neurol 2008; 21: 628–633.

54. Contreras-Vidal JL and Buch ER. Effects of Parkinson's disease on visuomotor adaptation. Exp Brain Res 2003; 150: 25–32.

55. Smith MA and Shadmehr R. Intact ability to learn internal models of arm dynamics in Huntington's disease but not cerebellar degeneration. J Neurophysiol 2005; 93: 2809–2821.

56. Weiner MJ, Hallett M and Funkenstein HH. Adaptation to lateral displacement of vision in patients with lesions of the central nervous system. Neurology 1983; 33: 766–772.

57. Brown RG and Jahanshahi M. Cognitive-motor dysfunction in Parkinson's disease. Eur Neurol 1996; 36 Suppl 1: 24–31.

58. Pieruccini-Faria F, Ehgoetz Martens, Kaylena A, Silveira CR, Jones JA and Almeida QJ. Interactions between cognitive and sensory load while planning and controlling complex gait adaptations in Parkinson's disease. BMC Neurol 2014; 14: 250.

59. Hely MA, Morris, John G L, Reid, Wayne G J and Trafficante R. Sydney Multicenter Study of Parkinson's disease: non-L-dopa-responsive problems dominate at 15 years. Mov. Disord. 2005; 20: 190–199.